CW00518510

The Best Cookbo
Diabetes

Simple Recipes for the Entire Family.
Easy and Quick Preparations for Busy
People with Diabetes

By

Tiara Crocker

© Copyright 2021 By Tiara Crocker — All Rights Reserved.

This document is geared towards providing exact and reliable information in regards to the topic and issue covered. The publication is sold with the idea that the publisher is not required to render accounting, officially permitted, or otherwise, qualified services. If advice is necessary, legal or professional, a practiced individual in the profession should be ordered.

From a Declaration of Principles which was accepted and approved equally by a Committee of the American Bar Association and a Committee of Publishers and Associations.

In no way is it legal to reproduce, duplicate, or transmit any part of this document in either electronic means or in printed format. Recording of this publication is strictly prohibited and any storage of this document is not allowed unless with written permission from the publisher. All rights reserved.

The information provided herein is stated to be truthful and consistent, in that any liability, in terms of inattention or otherwise, by any usage or abuse of any policies, processes, or directions contained within is the solitary and utter responsibility of the recipient reader. Under no circumstances will any legal responsibility or blame be held against the publisher for any reparation, damages, or monetary loss due to the information herein, either directly or indirectly.

Respective authors own all copyrights not held by the publisher.

The information herein is offered for informational purposes solely, and is universal as so. The presentation of the information is without contract or any type of guarantee assurance.

The trademarks that are used are without any consent, and the publication of the trademark is without permission or backing by the trademark owner. All trademarks and brands within this book are for clarifying purposes only and are the owned by the owners themselves, not affiliated with this document.

TABLE OF CONTENTS

INTRODUCTION

Are you tired of seeing ads on social networks about diets? Do you trust anyone who tells you that you can control Diabetes in an uncomplicated way?

Well, The Best Cookbook for the Diabetes came to change your life. Throughout this book, you will find unique and innovative ways to transform your diet and obtain many benefits for your life.

You can usually see information about miracle diets on almost all audiovisual platforms, however, this book contains the 50 must-have recipes that can help to control

Diabetes, boost the immune system and have a lot of fun while doing it.

Yes, you read that right, you can have fun and nutrition at the same time since each recipe is practical, creative and delicious.

In this book you will find:

1. Snacks to recover energy, snacks with a high level of protein and incredible desserts.

2. Healthy and delicious dishes.

3. Unique flavors that you must try.

4. Awesome salads

Start your new life, today is the perfect day to do it!

CHAPTER 1 BREAKFAST RECIPES

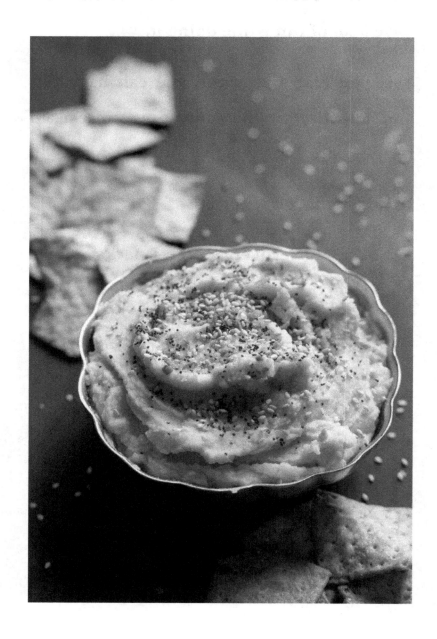

1.1 Everything Bagel with Hummus

(**Prep. time:** 10 min. | **Servings:** 2 | **Difficulty:** easy)

Serving size: 1 slice

Per serving: Kcal 213, Fat 11.6g, Net Carbs 19.5g, Proteins 6.8g

Ingredients

- 2 pieces gluten-free toasted bread

- 1 soft boiled egg, halved

- 2 tsp. Everything Bagel Spice (if not available then look at the recipe below after the instructions)

- 6 tbsp. hummus

- A pinch of paprika

- Olive oil

If you cannot find the spice then use this recipe to make your own:

- 1 tbsp. sesame seeds

- ½ tsp. powdered garlic

- ½ tsp. poppy seeds

- ¼ tsp. sea salt, fine

- 1 tbsp. dried minced onion

- 1 tsp. minced dried garlic

- ½ tsp. sea salt, coarse

Directions

1. Spread 3 tbsp. hummus on the bread slices.

2. Add a half egg to the slices and add the 'Everything Bagel' on top.

3. Add the paprika and olive oil then serve.

1.2 Mexican Scramble

You may not be able to eat this Mexican inspired recipe with your hands like a tortilla wrap, but trust me — you will enjoy every bite!

(Prep. time: 45 min. | **Servings:** 4 | **Difficulty:** medium)

Serving size: 1 slice

Per serving: Kcal 227, Fat 4.8g, Net Carbs 21.8g, Proteins 23.8g

Ingredients

- 4 corn tortillas (6-inches)

- 2 links cooked and sliced chicken sausages

- 1 medium halved and sliced onion

- 1 cup red bell pepper, cut into bite-size strips

- 1 fresh jalapeño chili pepper or poblano, chopped and seeded

- 2 cups frozen/refrigerated egg product, thawed, or 8 eggs, beaten lightly

- ⅛ tsp. salt

- ¼ cup queso fresco, crumbled or reduced-fat Monterey Jack cheese, grated (1-oz.)

- Fresh cilantro sprigs (optional)

- Fresh jalapeño chili pepper slices (optional)

Directions

1. Heat oven to 400°F. Bake the corn tortillas for 7 to 8 minutes or until they are crisp. Break into coarse pieces and set aside.

2. Cook sausage, onion, chili pepper, and bell pepper in a large pan over medium heat for around 6 minutes, until the sausage is browned and vegetables are cooked.

3. Add salt, eggs, Monterey Jack, and the tortilla pieces. Cook without stirring, till the mix starts to set around the edges and on the bottom. With a large spoon, lift and fold the egg mixture so that the uncooked mixture goes underneath. Continue cooking for 2 to 3 minutes, until it is cooked through but still moist and glossy. Then remove from stove. Garnish with fresh jalapeño pepper and fresh cilantro before serving.

1.3 Mushroom and Sausage Breakfast Casserole

(**Prep. time:** 3 hrs. 25 min. | **Servings:** 6 | **Difficulty:** medium)

Serving size: 1 piece

Per serving: Kcal 285, Fat 11.5g, Net Carbs 25g, Proteins 21.8g

Ingredients

- 2 tsp. olive oil

- 1 medium green or red chopped sweet pepper

- 1 cup sliced button mushrooms or fresh cremini

- 1 chopped medium onion

- 6 oz. thinly sliced smoked turkey sausage

- 8 oz. baguette-style bread, whole-grain, cut to cubes

- ½ cup shredded, cheddar or reduced-fat Swiss cheese

- 3 whites eggs

- 4 eggs

- 1 tsp. crushed dried oregano

- 2 cups milk, fat-free

Directions

1. Heat oil in a big pan. Add mushrooms, onions, and sweet pepper to the pan; cook for 5 minutes on medium heat, until they are tender, stir frequently.

2. Take a 2-quart rectangle baking dish and lightly grease it. Arrange one-half of the bread cubes, layering them evenly on the dish. Top the bread with half the mushroom mix, half of the sausage, and half of the cheese. Make several layers by repeating these steps.

3. Take a bowl and mix eggs, milk, egg whites, and oregano with a whisk. Pour this over the layered dish, slowly. Press it down lightly using the backside of a big spoon. Cover it and chill it for 2 hours or for a day.

4. Preheat your oven to 350°F. Uncover the casserole, and bake it for 50 minutes or till it is set and browned lightly on the top (There may be some liquid egg in the center of the casserole). Let it stand for 10 minutes before you serve it (the egg liquid will set at this point). Cut the casserole into 6 equal pieces.

1.4 Quick Cinnamon Roll Oats

These oats are prepared the night before, and take 5 minutes to prep

(**Prep. time:** 5 min. | **Servings:** 5 | **Difficulty:** easy)

Serving size: $^2/3$ cup

Per serving: Kcal 197, Fat 4g, Net Carbs 35g, Proteins 5g

Ingredients

- 2 ½ cup rolled oats

- 5 tsp. stevia

- 2 ½ cups non-dairy unsweetened milk

- 2 ½ tsp. vanilla extract

- ½ tsp. salt

- 1 ¼ tsp. ground cinnamon

Directions

1. Stir milk, oats, stevia, salt, cinnamon, and vanilla in a big bowl.

2. Pour the mixture into five 8-oz. jars.

3. Put on the lids and put it in the fridge the night before or for 5 days.

1.5 Banana and Peanut Butter Cinnamon Toast

(**Prep. time:** 5min. | **Servings:** 1 | **Difficulty**: easy)

Serving size: 1 toast

Per serving: Kcal 266, Fat 9.3g, Net Carbs 38g, Proteins 8g

Ingredients

- 1 small sliced banana
- 1 slice toasted bread (whole wheat)
- 1 tbsp. peanut butter
- Cinnamon powder to taste

Directions

1. Spread peanut butter on toast and top it with slices of banana.

2. Sprinkle it with cinnamon, according to taste.

CHAPTER 2 SNACKS

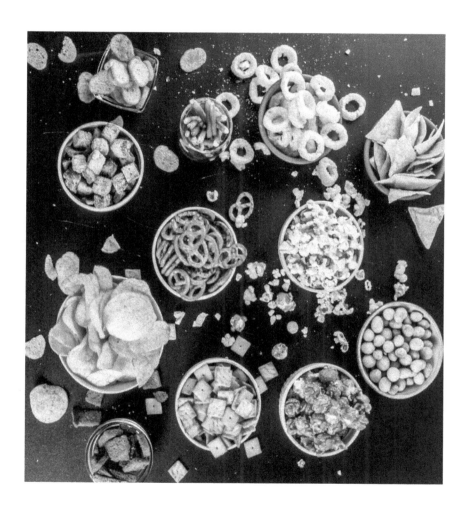

2.1 Six Cups Microwave Popcorn

Popcorn provides a snack anytime you want with a limited number of calories. Many types of microwaves popcorns have just 100 calories per 6 cups. It also has a strong fiber material, which will help you remain full longer.

2.2 Mini Quesadilla

Cheese quesadillas are an unexpected entry in a low-calorie snack list but try this recipe: scattered an oz. of grated no-fat cheddar cheese over a tortilla of corn. Fold it and microwave for 30 seconds. This tasty and quick snack has only 100 calories and 1.3 g of fat.

2.3 Three Crackers with Cheese

Choose whole-grain, low-fat crackers for this classic snack. Its fiber will keep you full in between meals, and the cheese gives a source of Proteins and calcium. To remain under 100 calories, use one slice of low-fat cheese and split it over three crackers.

2.4 Healthy cantaloupe snack

Cottage Cheese and Cantaloupe

Cottage cheese is a nutrition king, containing 14 g in ½ cup. Food high in fiber will help you remain full longer. Savor cottage cheese with low fat as ii or with a wedge of the fruit. A tiny cantaloupe wedge takes overall calories to 100.

2.5 Fourteen Almonds

When you're on the move, and the munchies hit, there are a few items handier than the nuts. You will consume 14 almonds without needing to touch the 100 calorie mark. Furthermore, they are high in Proteins and nutrition, which tend to hold hunger at bay.

2.6 Six Whole-Grain Pretzel Sticks

The pretzels are just as good for anyone who doesn't want nuts while you're on the move. Only have six whole-wheat pretzel sticks to stay within 100 calories. This snack is free from cholesterol, low in sugar and fat, and contains more than three grams of fiber to help you tide over.

2.7 Baked Apple

Apples are always one of the healthiest treats available, and this classic favorite has lots of ways to add a twist. Baked apples are a joy to eat – they taste sweet, plus they have the same antioxidants and fiber as their fresh contemporaries. You can also scatter cinnamon on top with no calories to add.

2.8 Cheese-Stuffed Pita Pocket

Here's one snack that's easy to create, and you get the pleasure of chewing on a sandwich. Take a pita pocket of whole-grain and fill it with ½ oz. skimmed ricotta cheese. The Proteins and fiber can help keep you full, and the entire snack contains less than a gram of saturated fat.

CHAPTER 3 SALADS RECIPES

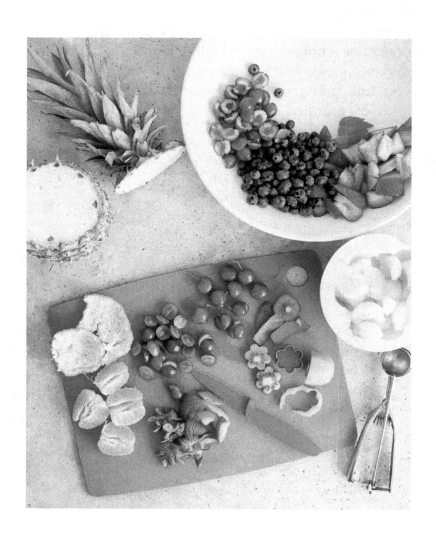

3.1 Summery Fruit Salad

(**Prep. time:** 30 min. | **Servings:** 4 | **Difficulty:** medium)

Serving size: 1 cup

Per serving: Calories: 260, fats: 7g, Carbs: 23g, Proteins: 24g

Ingredients

- ½ cup fresh blueberries

- ½ cup fresh blackberries

- ½ cup fresh raspberries

- ½ cup hulled and sliced fresh strawberries

- 2 medium size thinly sliced ripe peaches

- 1 cup seedless grapes

- 2 tbsp. lime juice, fresh

- 2 tbsp. Splenda o Stevia

Directions

1. Merge the fruit into a big tub. Blend in the sugar substitute and the lime juice.

2. Apply to the fruit mixture and stir to combine.

3. Enable the fruit salad to stand before serving for 20 minutes to allow the flavors to mix.

3.2 Spinach Salad and Flaxseed Lemon

Dressings on Salmon

Salmon is at the forefront of excellent and nutritious fish. Filled with beneficial fats and Omega-3 fatty acids, eating this tasty fish only a few days a week can't go wrong. This salad places salmon on top of a spinach bed with lemon flaxseed seasoning as its exquisite best style. It's guaranteed to be a success every day or night.

(Prep. time: | **Servings:** 4 to 6 | **Difficulty:** medium)

Serving size: ¼ of the recipe

Per serving: Kcal: 239, Fats: 15g, Carbs: 6g, Proteins: 20g

Ingredients

- 12 oz. grilled salmon
- 1c. water
- 3 cups fresh spinach
- 1 cup lemon juice
- 1 cup sliced cucumbers
- 3 garlic cloves, crushed
- ½ cup, sliced red onion
- 2 tbsp. oregano
- 4 tbsp. flax seeds
- 1/3 tsp. black pepper
- Stevia to taste

Directions

1. Bake or barbecue the salmon at 350°F until cooked.

2. Wash spinach and rinse. Toss the spinach in a large bowl with cucumbers and red onion. Combine dressing ingredients in a medium bowl.

3. Place the spinach salad on the plates and finish with the salmon. Sprinkle with dressings.

3.3 Easy Taco Salad

Taco salad is like tacos but much simpler to consume with even fewer calories. This salad will give you an additional boost of Proteins to keep your blood sugar steady, two portions of your veggies, and a pleasing crisp

(**Prep. time:** 30 min. | **Serves:** 6 | **Difficulty:** easy)

Serving size: 1 ½ cup

Per serving: Kcal: 330, Fats: 7g, Proteins: 21g, Carbs: 45g

Ingredients

- 1 lb. drained and cooked ground beef

- 1 Packet Taco Seasoning

- 1 cup diced tomato

- 1 cup cheddar cheese

- 1 cup grated carrots

- 1 bag crushed tortilla chips

- 1 sliced red onion

- 6 cups shredded lettuce

- 2 cups salsa

Directions

1. Wash and Brown ground beef.

2. Add taco salt as indicated on the box.

3. In a big bowl, place lettuce and throw in vegetables, tomatoes, cheese and onion.

4. Add cooled ground beef and crushed tortilla chips.

5. Cover with salsa or a low-fat salad sauce you like.

3.4 BBQ Chicken on a Bed of Spring Greens

To make a delicious dinner out of last night's BBQ, mix it with spring greens and veggies and a light vinaigrette.

(Prep. time: 10 min. | **Servings:** 2 | **Difficulty:** easy)

Serving size: 1 plate

Per serving: Kcal: 210, Fats: 4.5g, Carbs: 4g, Proteins: 21g

Ingredients

- ¼ sliced barbecue chicken breasts

- 2 cups spring greens

- ¼ sliced red onion

Directions

1. Toss Greens with onion and lay on a plate.

2. Top with barbecue chicken.

3. Drizzle with your favorite dressing or a light vinaigrette.

3.5 Chickpeas and Faro Salad

Vegetarian People who have diabetes ought to look for healthy Proteins sources. Faro is a delicious grain of Proteins and full of fiber that can add nutrition to your salad. The flavor of the meal is rather nutty, not smoky. This is a delicious salad inspired by the Caribbean.

(Prep. time: 30 min. │**Serves:** 3 to 4│**Difficulty:** medium)

Serving size: 2 cups

Per serving: Kcal: 241, Fats: 6.5g, Carbs: 39g, Proteins: 9.1g

Ingredients

- 3 cups faro grain

- ½ cup cool and cooked tahini

- 2 Roma Tomatoes, chopped

- ½ cup water

- 1 thinly sliced cucumber

- ¼ cup lemon juice

- ¼ bunch fresh parsley

- 2 garlic cloves, crushed

- 4 cups spring greens

- ½ tsp. cumin

- 1 can chick peas

- ¼ tsp. cayenne pepper

- ½ tsp. salt

Directions

1. In a wide bowl, throw the spring grass, onions, parsley, cucumber, and chickpeas

2. Mix dressing ingredients together in a medium bowl and drizzle over lettuce, then toss again.

3. Divide the salad over the plates and finish with the grain Faro. Even chickpeas can be marinated overnight in the sauce if desired.

3.6 Black Bean Salad and Quinoa

This Black Bean and Quinoa Salad is an easy-to-use recipe that you can use for packed lunches or quick meals all week long. It's filled with a maximum supply of plant-based nutrition, and is usually gluten-free, too!

(**Prep. time:** 15 min. │**Servings:** 2 to 3 │**difficulty:** medium)

Serving size: 1/3 of the recipe

Per serving: Kcal: 136 Fats: 4g, Carbs: 15g, Proteins: 20g

Ingredients

- 1 ½ cup quinoa

- 5 tbsp. lime juice

- 1 ½ cup cooked black beans

- 1 tsp. salt

- 1 ½ cup corn

- ¼ tsp. cumin

- 1 ½ tbsp. red-wine vinegar

- $^1/_3$ cup olive oil

- ¾ cup finely chopped bell pepper

- 2 jalapeno peppers

Directions

1. Well, clean the quinoa and wash. Simmer in salted water for 10 minutes. Don't overcook them. Drain it and fluff it with a pick.

2. Place the strainer over a boiling water pot and let steam for another 10 minutes. Toss the red wine vinegar with the black beans and apply the salt and pepper. Take quinoa off the stove and add it to a large dish.

3. Toss in a combination of maize, rice, tomatoes, and bell pepper. Mix coating ingredients into a separate bowl.

CHAPTER 4 SOUPS & STEWS

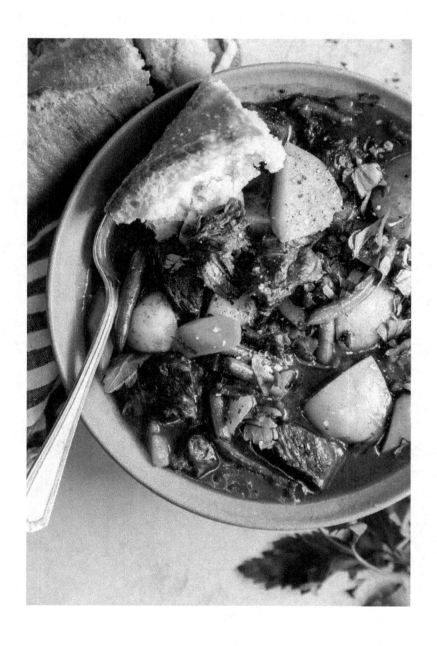

4.1 Classic Beef Stew

(**Prep. time:** 2 hrs. | **Servings:** 6 | **Difficulty:** medium)

Serving size: 1 cup

Per serving: Kcal 250, Fat 7g, Carbs 24g, Proteins 25g

Ingredients

- 2 tbsp. all-purpose flour or whole-wheat pastry flour

- 1 tbsp. Italian seasoning

- 3 tbsp. olive oil

- 2 lbs. top round (cut into ¾-inch cubes)

- 1 ½ lbs. cremini mushrooms (cleaned, stemmed & quartered)

- 4 cup low sodium chicken broth

- 1 large onion, chopped

- 1 garlic clove, minced

- Large russet potatoes 2

- 3 medium carrots

- 1 cup frozen peas

- 1 tbsp. fresh thyme, minced

- 1 tbsp. red wine vinegar

- ½ tsp. freshly ground black pepper

Directions

1. The all-purpose flour is mixed with Italian seasoning. Heat up the olive oil over moderate flame in a big Dutch oven. In the flour mixture, dredge the beef cubes gently and add the beef, in batches to maintain the beef in one layer until well browned on either side.

2. Take the beef out of the saucepan and deglaze with ¼ cup of chicken broth. Add the mushrooms, and sauté until well browned for around 4 minutes. Remove mushrooms from the saucepan and deglaze with a full ¼ cup of broth. Add the garlic and onions, and sauté for four minutes. Transfer the beef to the pot, add remaining broth of chicken and bring to a simmer. Cover partly, reduce heat to simmer, and cook for 45 min., stirring periodically.

3. Peel the potatoes and cut them into ¾ "bits. Cut carrots into ½ "bits. Add the potatoes and carrots to the stew & cook for an additional 45 minutes or until veggies are soft. Add reserved mushroom, peas, and thyme. Red wine vinegar & black pepper are for seasoning.

4.2 Easy Cream of Tomato Soup

(**Prep. time:** 35 min. | **Servings:** 12 | **Difficulty:** medium)

Serving size: 1 cup

Per serving: Cal 94, Fat 2g, Carbs 13g, Proteins 7g

Ingredients

- 1 tbsp. reduced-fat margarine

- 1 tbsp. canola oil

- 1 finely chopped medium onion

- ½ tsp. dried thyme, crushed

- ¼ tsp. dried oregano, crushed

- 5 cups no-salt-added canned chicken broth

- 3 cans no-salt-added diced tomatoes with the juice of 14.5 oz.

- Optional: pinch of cayenne pepper

- Optional: salt

- Freshly ground pepper to taste

- 2 cans of evaporated skim milk of 12 oz.

Directions

1. Heat margarine and oil in a heavy soup pot over medium-low flame.

2. Add onion and cook until the onion is really limp (about ten min.), stirring regularly, and taking note not to make the onion brown.

3. Add tomatoes with their juice, thyme, oregano, and chicken broth. Bring to a boil; minimize heat to low, and simmer for 20 min., partially covered.

4. Taste soup, add salt and cayenne (if used) and pepper to taste.

5. Stir in evaporated milk and heat. Do not make the mixture boil.

4.3 Cauliflower Almond Soup – Stack's Holiday Favorite

(**Prep. time**: 10 hrs. 30 min. | **Servings:** 4 | **Difficulty:** medium)

Serving size: ¼ of recipe

Per serving: Kcal 195, Fat 14g, Carbs 14g, Proteins 7g

Ingredients

- 2 tbsp. almond oil
- 2 stalks celery, chopped celery
- ½ cup sliced leek, white & light green portions
- ¾ tsp. kosher salt
- 4 cups cauliflower head, cut to florets
- 1-quart chicken broth, low sodium
- ¼ tsp. ground fresh black pepper
- ¼ tsp. ground nutmeg
- ¾ cup cashew-almond cream
- ¼ cup parsley, chopped
- ½ cups toasted sliced almonds

Directions

1. Heat almond oil over medium heat in a big soup pot. Put the celery, and cook before softening starts. Add leak and begin cooking until all vegetables are tender.

2. Steam some cauliflower and put aside for garnishing. In the vegetable mixture incorporate the cauliflower that is left, broth, pepper, nutmeg, and salt and bring it to boil. Simmer for about 10 min., till the cauliflower is tender.

3. Puree the soup using a food processor or blender. Add the cashew-almond cream and stir. Garnish each soup bowl with 1 parsley tbsp., 2 almond tablespoons, and some saved cauliflower florets.

4.4 Easy Chicken, Spinach, and Wild Rice Soup

(**Prep. time:** 15 min.| **Servings:** 6-7 | **Difficulty:** medium)

Serving size: 1 cup

Per serving: Cal 256, Fat 7g, Carbs 28g, Proteins 22g

Ingredients

- 1 can reduced-sodium chicken broth

- 1 ¾ cups chopped carrots

- 2 cans reduced-fat reduced-sodium condensed cream of chicken soup

- 2 cups cooked wild rice

- 1 tsp. dried thyme

- ¼ tsp. dried sage

- ¼ tsp. black pepper

- 2 cups chopped baby spinach

- 1 ½ cups chopped cooked chicken

- ½ cup fat-free half-and-half or fat-free (skim) milk

- A pinch of sugar substitute

Directions

1. Bring the broth to a boil over medium to high heat in a wide saucepan.

2. Add carrots, and cook for 10 minutes.

3. To saucepan, add broth, sugar subtitute, thyme, sage and pepper; carry to a boil.

4. Add lettuce, meat, and half-and-a-half; cook and mix for 2 min., or until heated.

4.5 Green pesto minestrone

(**Prep. time:** 25 min. | **Servings:** 4 | **Difficulty:** medium)

Serving size: 1 cup

Per serving: Kcal 334, Fat 17g, Carbs 24g, Proteins 19g

Ingredients

- 2 tbsp. olive oil

- 1 large onion finely chopped

- 2 celery sticks finely chopped

- Vegetable stock 1.4l

- Zest and juice of 2 lemon

- Orzo 170g

- Frozen peas 120g

- Frozen spinach 250g

- Pesto 50g

- Garlic flatbreads to serve (optional)

- Grated parmesan 60g

Directions

1. Heat the oil in a big saucepan, add the onions, celery as well as a pinch of salt, then fry until soft for 8 minutes. Stir in the stock with lemon zest and juice, and season. Add the orzo and cook for 5 minutes then add the peas & spinach and cook for another 5 minutes. Swirl the pesto and season.

2. If used, heat the flatbreads according to box directions. Ladle the soup in bowls generously, then top with parmesan. Serve to dip, with the flat-bread.

CHAPTER 5 POULTRY

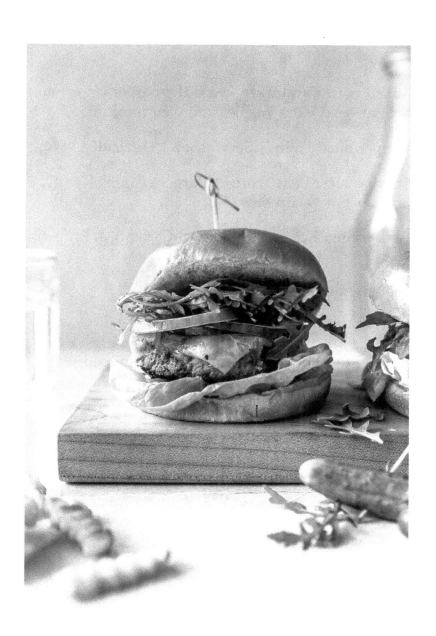

5.1 Zucchini and Turkey Burgers served with Corn on Cob

Mixed with lean turkey keeps the burgers moist and help to sneak extra veggies into your mealtime.

(**Prep. time:** 35 min. | **Servings:** 2 | **Difficulty:** easy)

Serving size: ½ ear corn+1 Burger (1 bun, 1 patty, 2 tsp. sauce) + ¼ cup slaw

Per serving: Kcal: 446, Fats: 19g, Carbs: 37g, Proteins: 21g

Ingredients

- 1 ¼ cups red cabbage, thinly sliced
- 2 tbsp. jalapeño pepper, finely chopped
- 1 tbsp. lime juice
- 1 tbsp. canola oil, plus ½ tsp., divided
- 1 tbsp. salt
- 2 tsp. mayonnaise,
- 2 tsp. low-fat plain yogurt
- ¾ tsp. chili powder
- 1 ear corn, husked and halved

- turkey breast (99% Lean), 5 oz. ground

- ½ cup zucchini, shredded

- 3 tbsp. panko breadcrumbs

- 3 tbsp. red/yellow onion, finely chopped

- ½ tsp. ground cumin

- ⅛ tsp. ground pepper

- 1 oz. pepper jack cheese

- 2 whole-wheat hamburger rolls, split and toasted

Directions

1. Heat the oven grill to medium-high. Mix cabbage, lime juice, jalapeño, 1 tbsp. Oil, and around ⅛ tsp. Salt in a medium mixing bowl. Cool ½ cup of the slaw in the fridge.

2. in a small tub, mix mayo, yogurt, and chili powder. Apply the remaining ½ tsp. of oil on the corn.

3. Combine the zucchini, turkey panko crumbs, the onion, pepper, cumin, and ⅛ tsp. 1 Salt left in a medium mixing bowl. Shape the two ¾-inch thick patties from this mixture.

4. Apply Grill rack with oil. Grill the corn, rotating it periodically, for 6 to 10 minutes, till some kernels sear a little and others are light brown. Meanwhile, BBQ the patties until cooked, an instant-read thermometer must register 165°F when inserted, cook for 4 to five min. on each side. Before the patties are cooked, coat them with slices of cheese and let it melt slightly.

5. Apply the paste of mayonnaise over the sliced buns of hamburger. The remaining slaw is divided between the buns. Put the patties on the buns and cover with the other half. Break the corn in two and serve half of it with each burger.

5.2 Chicken & Veggie Quesadilla

Make these easy quesadillas with cooked or canned chicken to save time. Using leftover cooked chicken or turkey will make it simpler still. Dice the veggies one day ahead for even quicker prep.

(**Prep. time:** 20 min. | **Servings:** 1 | **Difficulty:** easy)

Serving size: 1 Quesadilla

Per serving: Kcal: 436, Fats: 21g, Carbs: 32g, Proteins: 26g

Ingredients

- 2 tsp. canola oil

- ¼ cup onion, chopped

- ¼ cup red bell pepper, diced

- ¼ cup zucchini, diced

- 2 oz. cooked chicken, shredded

- 2 tbsp. frozen or fresh corn kernels

- Optional: 1 tbsp. fresh cilantro, chopped

- 1 (8-inch) whole-wheat tortilla

- 3 tbsp. pepper jack cheese, shredded

Directions

1. Heat oil on medium heat in a big skillet. Add the bell pepper, zucchini, and onion; cook, continually stirring until the veggies are tender, for about 3 to 4 min. Add the chicken and the corn; cook for around 1 minute until it is heated. Sprinkle in cilantro if you have it. Place the vegetables in a little bowl.

2. Put a tortilla on a chopping board. Sprinkle with 1 tbsp. Cheese on half of the tortilla, leaving a ½-inch edge. Cover with the mixture of vegetables and the remainder 2 tbsp. of cheese. Fold the tortilla in two.

3. Place the pan over medium heat. Cook the quesadilla until the tortilla is cooked has gotten a little color, and the cheese begins to melt, around 2 minutes per side.

4. Serve after cutting in three pieces.

5.3 Grilled Chicken with brown rice & Roasted Cauliflower

(**Prep. time:** 20 min. | **Servings:** 2 | **Difficulty:** easy)

Serving size: half of the recipe

Per serving: Kcal: 543, Fats: 26g, Carbs: 44g, Proteins: 34g

Ingredient

- 10 oz. skinless, boneless, chicken thighs (about 3), cut into 6 pieces

- 2 tsp. olive oil

- 2 tsp. ground cinnamon

- ½ tsp. salt, plus ¼ tsp., divided

- 1 ½ cups cooked brown [wu1] rice

- 1 cup roasted cauliflower

- ⅔ cup roasted green peppers

- ⅔ cup roasted red peppers

- ¼ cup chicken broth/vegetable broth, low-sodium

- 2 tsp. lemon juice, plus wedges for serving

- ¼ cup fresh mint leaves

- 1 tbsp. pine nuts, toasted

Directions

1. Heat a large frying pan or a grill pan on medium-high heat. Brush oil on chicken. Sprinkle cinnamon and ⅛ tsp. of salt on the chicken. Cook the chicken turning it occasionally until the chicken is golden brown and is thoroughly cooked for about 10 minutes.

2. Meanwhile, in a medium-sized saucepan, combine brown rice, green / red peppers, cauliflower, lemon juice, broth, and the remaining ¼ tsp. Salt. Cover and cook on med. Heat for about 8 minutes or until heated through.

3. Serve the cooked chicken over the rice and vegetables. Garnish with mint leaves and pine nuts. Serve with cut lemon wedges, if desired.

5.4 Healthy Turkey Meatballs (Without Breadcrumbs)

These Healthy Turkey Meatballs without Breadcrumbs are juicy little Proteins bombs that are packed with flavor! They're super easy to make and ready in just 40 minutes.

(**Prep. time:** 40 min. | **Servings:** 5 | **Difficulty:** easy)

Serving size: 3 meatballs

Per serving: Kcal: 183, Fats: 3g, Carbs: 9g, Proteins: 30g

Ingredients

- 20 oz. ground turkey

- 3.5 oz. fresh/frozen spinach

- ¼ cup oats

- 2 egg whites

- 2 sticks celery

- 3 garlic cloves

- ½ bell pepper, green

- ½ red onion

- ½ cup parsley

- ½ tsp. cumin

- 1 tsp. mustard powder

- 1 tsp. thyme

- ½ tsp. turmeric

- ½ tsp. chipotle pepper

- 1 tsp. salt

- Pinch of pepper

Directions

1. Heat the oven to 175°C (350°F).

2. Chop the garlic, celery, and onion very finely, then add them to a large mixing bowl.

3. Add the egg meat, whites, spices, and oats, to the bowl and mix evenly. Make sure spices and oats are not clumped in the mix.

4. Chop all the veggies into dime-sized pieces.

5. Add them to the bowl and mix everything till well-combined.

6. Line parchment paper on a baking sheet.

7. Make 15 balls of the turkey mixture (about the size of golf balls) and place them on the baking sheet.

8. Bake for about 25 minutes, or until cooked through.

5.5 Chicken Nuggets

These golden chicken nuggets are so quick and easy to make. Everyone loves them. Its versatile seasoning can be used to cook chicken breasts also. Load them on country bread with mayo and salad veggies to make delicious sandwiches.

(Prep. time: 30 min. | **Servings:** 8 | **Difficulty:** easy)

Serving size: 3 oz. cooked chicken

Kcal: 212, Fats: 10g, Carbs: 6g, Proteins: 24g

Ingredients

- 1 cup all-purpose flour
- 4 tsp. seasoned salt
- 1 tsp. poultry seasoning
- 1 tsp. ground mustard
- 1 tsp. paprika
- ½ tsp. pepper
- 2 lb. chicken breasts, skinless and boneless
- ¼ cup canola oil

Directions

1. In a large mixing dish, combine the first six ingredients.

1. 2.beat with a mallet to Flatten chicken to a. thickness of half an inch, then cut into one and a half-inch Pieces.

2. Add a few pieces of chicken to the mixing dish, and turn them over to coat every piece.

3. In a large frying pan, cook chicken in oil in small batches for 6 to 8 min. Or until meat is cooked.

CHAPTER 6 FISH AND SEAFOOD

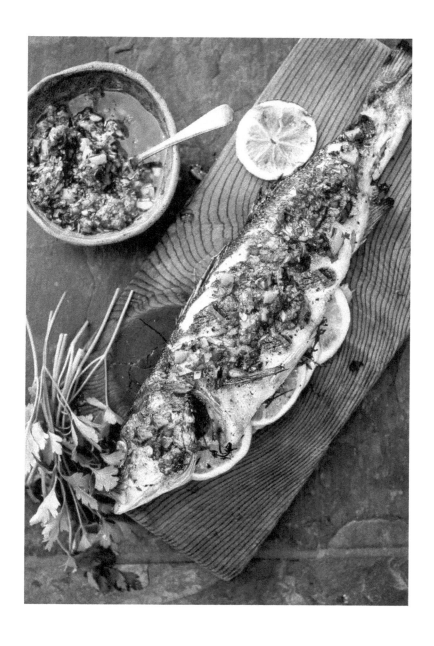

6.1 Herby Mediterranean Fish with Wilted Greens & Mushrooms

(**Prep. time:** 25 min. | **Servings:** 4 | **Difficulty:** medium)

Serving size: 1 piece fish + ½ cup Vegetables

Per serving: Cal 214, Fat 11g, Carbs 11g, Proteins 18g

Ingredients

- 3 tbsp. olive oil

- ½ large sweet onion, sliced

- 3 cups cremini mushrooms, sliced

- 2 garlic cloves, sliced

- 4 cups chopped kale

- 1 medium tomato, diced

- 2 tsp. Mediterranean Herb Mix

- 1 tbsp. lemon juice

- ½ tsp. salt

- ½ tsp. ground pepper

- 4 (4 oz.) cod, sole, or tilapia fillets

- Chopped fresh parsley, for garnishing

Directions:

1. Heat 1 tbsp. oil over medium heat in a wide saucepan. Transfer onion; cook for 3 to 4 minutes, stirring periodically, until translucent.

2. Add mushrooms and garlic; cook for 4 to 6 minutes, stirring regularly, before the mushrooms release their liquid and start brown.

3. Add the tomatoes, kale, and 1 tsp. Herbal combination. Cook, stirring regularly, for 5 to 7 minutes, until the kale wilts and the mushrooms are soft. Stir in lemon juice, salt & pepper ¼ tsp. each. Remove from heat, cover and keep warm.

4. Brush the remaining 1 tsp. herb mix on fish and ¼ tsp. salt and pepper. Heat the remaining 2 tablespoons. Oil over medium to high heat in a large, non-stick skillet. Add the fish & cook until the flesh becomes opaque, depending on thickness, 2 to 4 min. per side. Place the fish on four plates or a serving platter.

5. Cover with the vegetables and surround the fish; sprinkle with parsley if necessary.

6.2 Provençal Fish Fillets

(**Prep. time:** 25 min. | **Servings:** 4 | **Difficulty:** medium)

Serving size: 1 serving

Per serving: Kcal 161, Fat 5.2g, Carbs 7.2g, Proteins 21.4g

Ingredients

- 1 tbsp. olive oil

- 4 (4 oz.) frozen or fresh skinless cod, Pollock, or catfish 0.5 to 1 inch in thickness

- 1 medium onion thinly sliced

- 2 garlic cloves, minced

- 1 can tomatoes, chopped and drained tomatoes

- 2 tsp. fresh thyme, chopped, or ½ tsp. dried & crushed

- 8 pitted ripe olives, halved ripe

- 1 tsp. capers, drained

- Fresh sprigs of thyme, if desired

Directions

1. If frozen, thaw fish. Rinse the fish with paper towels; pat dry. Put aside.

2. Boil oil over medium heat in a shallow saucepan. Add garlic and onion; fry, stirring regularly, for around 5 min. or till tender. Add tomatoes, olives, thyme, and capers. Boil; reduce to medium heat. Simmer for approximately 10 minutes, uncovered, or till much of the fluid has been evaporated.

3. Meanwhile, broiler preheat. Measure Fish Thickness. Put fish in a broiler pan on the greased unheated rack, tucking under the thin edges. Then broil 3–4 inches away from heat for about 4–6 min. per 0.5 inches thick fish, turn the fish just once if they are one inch wide.

4. Serve the prepared sauce with the fillet, and garnish with sprigs of fresh thyme if needed.

6.3 Italian Fish Stew

(**Prep. time:** 30 min. | **Servings:** 4 | **Difficulty:** medium)

Serving size: 4 oz. salmon + 1 ¼ cup vegetables + 2 tsp. Sauce

Per serving: Cal 165, Fat 4g, Carbs 12g, Proteins 19g

Ingredients

- ¹/₃ cup chopped onion

- 8 oz. fresh or frozen skinless cod or sea bass fillets

- 6 oz. fresh or frozen medium shrimp, peeled and deveined

- 2 stalks sliced celery

- ½ tsp. garlic, minced

- 2 tsp. olive oil

- 1 cup reduced-sodium chicken broth

- ¼ cup dry white wine or reduced-sodium chicken broth

- 1 can tomatoes no-salt-added drained diced

- 1 can no-salt-added tomato sauce

- 1 tsp. dried oregano, crushed

- ¼ tsp. salt

- ⅛ tsp. ground black pepper

- 1 tbsp. fresh parsley

Directions:

1. Thaw the shrimp and the fish, if frozen. Rinse fish and shrimp; pat dry with towels made from paper.

2. Cut the fish into pieces of 1-½ inch. Cut shrimps lengthwise in half. Fish and shrimp are covered and chilled until required.

3. Cook the onion, celery, and garlic in a large saucepan in hot oil until tender. Stir in 1 cup of broth and wine, slowly. Bring to boil; minimize flame. Simmer down for 5 min., uncovered.

4. Add tomatoes, tomato sauce, oregano, salt and pepper. Return to boiling; reduce fire. Cover then cook for five minutes.

5. Mix the fish and shrimp gently. Return solely to boil; minimize heat to minimum. Cover and simmer for 3 to 5 minutes or until the fish flakes with a fork and shrimp quickly become opaque. Parsley to sprinkle with.

6.4 Jalapeño shrimp veggie bake

(**Prep. time:** 55 min. | **Servings:** 4 | **Difficulty:** easy)

Serving size: ¼ of recipe

Per serving: Cal 240, Fat 9g, Carbs 8g, Proteins 20g

Ingredients

- 10–15 medium shrimp
- ¼ cup red onion, sliced
- 1 large tomato, sliced
- 2 yellow squash/zucchini
- 1 jalapeno, sliced and deseeded
- ¹/₃ cup cream or coconut cream
- 3 eggs
- 1 tbsp. melted butter
- 2 garlic cloves
- 2 tbsp. gluten-free starch or ¼ cup gluten-free flour
- Sea salt & black pepper to taste
- ¹/₃ – ½ cup grated parmesan or nutritional yeast for a dairy-free option

- ½ tsp. chili pepper flakes

- Cilantro & chili flakes for toppings and garnishing

Directions

1. First, make sure the shrimp has been peeled and thawed out. Preheat to 350°F

2. Next, see to it that all the vegetables are cut. If you want more spice to the bowl, first, the onion in the pan (until fragrant) will be lightly brown (dry sauté). Then gently spray or grease your pan and evenly layer the majority of the vegetables into baking dish or pan. Place the shrimp on top of the veggie layers or mix them together.

3. Combine cream, garlic, egg, starch, & butter, or oil, in a shallow bowl. Whisk till the mixture is smooth and yellow.

4. Pour this over your shrimp & vegetable dish uniformly. Sprinkle your sea salt & black pepper over a casserole dish accompanied, thinly, by your grated parmesan.

5. Garnishing with red pepper flakes.

6. Put it in the oven and bake for 35–45 minutes at 350°F, depending on your oven. Just make sure your shrimp is fried, and your vegetables are tender and good. Check to see progress around 25–30 minutes. While frying, the shrimp would shrink.

6.5 Tuna Nicosia Salad

(**Prep. time:** 15 min. | **Servings:** 1 | **Difficulty:** easy)

Serving size: 1 bowl

Per serving: Kcal 405, Fat 13.1g, Net Carbs 12.2g, Proteins 39g

Ingredients

- 4 oz. ahi tuna steak

- 1 egg

- 3 oz. baby spinach

- 2 oz. green beans

- 1 ½ oz. broccoli

- ½ red bell pepper

- 3 ½ oz. cucumber

- 1 radish

- 3 large black olives

- 1 tsp. olive oil

- Handful of parsley

- 1 tsp. balsamic vinegar

- ½ tsp. Dijon mustard

- ½ tsp. pepper

Directions

1. Boil an egg, then put it aside to cool.

2. Steam beans and broccoli, then put back. 2-3 minutes with a little water in the microwave, or 3 minutes in a kettle of boiling water.

3. In a pan, heat a bit of oil over high heat. Season the tuna on both sides with pepper, then put it in the pan & cook each side for around 2 minutes.

4. Apply the spinach to the bowl or plate for salads.

5. Cut the bell pepper, cucumber, and egg into pieces of bite-size. Add it to the spinach.

6. Cut radish into slices and mix in the broccoli, beans and olives together. Add on top of the spinach salad.

7. Cut the tuna into slices and add it to the salad.

8. Mix the olive oil, balsamic vinegar, and mustard, salt and pepper together.

9. Cut the parsley, and add to the vinaigrette.

10. To drizzle the vinaigrette over the salad, use a spoon.

6.6 Grilled Fish with Buttery Lemon Parsley

(**Prep. time:** 20 min. | **Servings:** 6 | **Difficulty:** medium)

Serving size: 1 fish fillet with 1 tbsp. sauce

Per serving: Cal 211, Fat 7g, Carbs 2g, Proteins 33g

Ingredients

- 6 tbsp. yogurt-based diet margarine

- 3 tbsp. chopped fresh parsley

- 1 tsp. grated lemon peel

- ½ tsp. salt

- ½ tsp. dried rosemary

- 6 fish fillets such as grouper, snapper, or any lean white fish of 6 oz. each one

- 3 medium halved lemons

- Nonstick cooking spray

Directions

1. Coat the cold grid with the cooking spray. Ready the grill fit for direct cooking.

2. In a small container, mix the margarine, parsley, lemon peel, salt, and rosemary; set it aside.

3. Cover fish with spray for cooking.

4. Place them over high heat on the grid. Grill for 3 minutes, uncovered. Turn; grill 2 or 3 min. longer or until it becomes opaque in the center.

5. Squeeze 1 half lemon juice over each fillet to eat.

6. Top with parsley mixture.

CHAPTER 7 VEGETABLES RECIPES

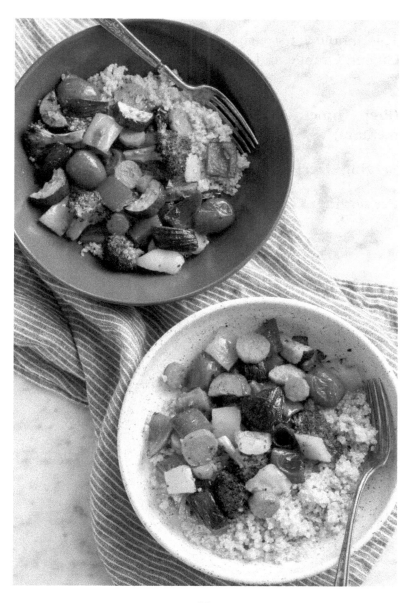

7.1 Spinach and White Beans with Ginger, Orange, and Sesame Dressing

This simple yet stylish Spinach and White Beans with Ginger, Orange and Sesame Seasoning will please all your guests!

(**Prep. time:** 30 min. | **Servings:** 4 | **Difficulty:** medium)

Serving size: ¼ of recipe

Per serving: Kcal: 68, Fats: 1g, Carbs: 13g, Proteins: 4g

Ingredients

- ¼ cup chicken broth, low sodium

- 8 cups baby spinach leaves

- ½ cup white beans, cooked

- ⅛ tsp. kosher salt

- ⅛ tsp. ground black pepper, fresh

- ¼ cup sesame, orange and ginger dressing

Directions

1. Over medium-high prepare, prepare a pan. Add the spinach and chicken broth. Let the spinach sag and the stock to decrease marginally.

2. To lessen the broth by at least half the amount, mix in the salt, beans, pepper, and cook.

3. Put in the mixture of spinach, whole beans, and ginger, sesame and orange. Season and enjoy it.

7.2 Spicy Chickpeas & Couscous

(**Prep. time:** 20 min. | **Servings:** 6 | **Difficulty:** easy)

Serving size: 1/6 of recipe

Per serving: Kcal: 226, Fats: 2g, Carbs: 2g, Proteins: 9g

Ingredients

- 1 can (about 14 oz.) vegetable broth

- 1 tsp. ground coriander

- ½ tsp. ground cardamom

- ½ tsp. turmeric

- ½ tsp. hot pepper sauce

- ¼ tsp. salt

- ⅛ tsp. ground cinnamon

- 1 cup carrots, match stick size

- 1 can (15 oz.) rinsed and drained, chickpeas

- 1 cup green peas, frozen

- 1 cup couscous, quick-cooking

- 2 tbsp. parsley or fresh mint, chopped

Directions

1. In a large saucepan, add vegetable broth, cardamom, coriander, turmeric, salt, pepper, and cinnamon; bring to boil over high heat. Stir in carrots; minimize heat and simmer for 5 minutes.

2. Add in the Chickpeas and green peas; return to a simmer. Simmer 2 minutes, without covering.

3. Add in couscous. Cover and take off from the heat. Let sit for 5 minutes, or before it absorbs the material. Scatter mint over it.

7.3 Broccoli & Cauliflower Stir-Fry

This vegetarian meal is simple to cook and full of fibers and taste!

(Prep. time: 35 min. | **Servings:** 2 | **Difficulty:** easy)

Serving size: ½ of recipe

Per serving: Kcal: 155, Fats: 8g, Carbs: 19g, Proteins: 6g

Ingredients

- 2 tomatoes, sun-dried (not packed in oil)
- 1 tbsp. soy sauce + 1 tsp. reduced-sodium
- 1 tbsp. vinegar of rice wine
- 1 tsp. sugar substitute (Splenda or truvia)
- 1 tsp. sesame oil, dark
- ⅛ tsp. flakes of red pepper
- 2 ¼ tsp. canola oil
- 1 garlic clove, finely chopped
- 2 cups cauliflower florets
- 2 cups broccoli florets
- 1/3 cup red or green bell pepper, thinly sliced

Directions

1. In a small tub, put the tomatoes; cover with hot water. Leave for 5 minutes. Drain and then cut finely. In the meantime, in a small cup, put together vinegar, soy sauce, sugar substitute, red pepper flakes and sesame oil.

2. Heat vegetable oil over medium-high heat in skillet or big, nonstick pan. Put garlic; fry and stir for 30 seconds. Add broccoli and cauliflower; fry and stir for 4 minutes; put in the tomatoes and the pepper bell; fry and stir for 1 minute, or until the vegetables are crispy

3. Add a mixture of soy sauce; continue cooking until heated. Instantly serve.

7.4 Grilled Veggie Pizza

Grilling the vegetables brings out their spicy flavors. Before using the cheese, sprinkle olives or pine nuts.

(**Prep. time:** 40 min.| **Servings:** 6| **Difficulty:** medium)

Serving size: 1 slice

Per serving: Kcal: 274, Fats: 11g, Carbs: 30g, Proteins: 17g

Ingredients

- Halved, fresh mushrooms

- 1 small zucchini, cut into ¼-inch slices

- 1 sliced sweet yellow pepper

- 1 small sweet red pepper, sliced

- 1 small onion, sliced

- 1 tbsp. white wine vinegar

- 1 tbsp. water

- 4 tsp. olive oil, divided

- 2 tsp. fresh basil, minced or ½ tsp. basil, dried

- ¼ tsp. salt

- ¼ tsp. pepper

- 12-inch whole-wheat pizza crust, thin and prebaked,1

- 1 can (8 oz.) pizza sauce

- 2 small chopped tomatoes

- 2 cups mozzarella cheese, shredded

Directions

1. Combine the zucchini, mushrooms, peppers, water, vinegar, onion, three teaspoons of oil and seasonings in a large tub. Move into a basket or barbecue wok. Grill, sealed, for 8-10 minutes over medium heat until soft, mixing one time.

2. Prepare barbeque for indirect fire.

3. Rub the crust with the excess oil; apply the pizza sauce to spread.

4. Grilled onions, tomatoes and cheese are added to the top.

5. Grill, keeping covered, for 10-12 minutes over indirect medium heat or until the sides are nicely browned, and cheese melts. Spin the pizza halfway through the cooking process to make sure the crust is properly browned.

7.5 Roasted Vegetable Strata

With the abundance of zucchini in the fall, this is an excellent recipe to use a little of what we've got. The hot, traditional breakfast dish, cheesy and delicious, is sure to delight you!

(**Prep. time:** 1 hr. 25 min. | **Servings:** 8 | **Difficulty:** hard)

Serving size: 1 piece

Per serving: Kcal: 349, Fats: 14g, Carbs: 40g, Proteins: 17g

Ingredients

- 3 large zucchini, halved lengthwise, cut into ¾-inch slices

- 1 each, medium range, yellow and red peppers, cut into 1-inch pieces

- 2 tbsp. olive oil

- 1 tsp. oregano, dried

- ½ tsp. salt

- ½ tsp. pepper

- ½ tsp. basil, dried

- 1 medium chopped tomato

- 1 loaf (1 pound) Italian bread, unsliced, crusted

- ½ cup cheddar cheese, shredded sharp

- ½ cup asiago cheese, shredded

- 6 large eggs

- 2 cups milk, fat-free

Directions

1. Preheat the oven to 400°F.

2. Shift to a 15x10x1-inch pan. Put in zucchini and peppers with oil and dressing. Roast for 25-30 minutes until soft, mixing often.

3. Mix in tomato and let it cool a little.

4. Trim the ends of the loaf; cut into 1-in loaf slices. In a greased 13x9-in. baking tray put half layer of each: bread, roasted cheeses and vegetables. Once again, repeat the layers. Stir the eggs and milk together; spread uniformly over the top. Refrigerate, sealed, overnight or 6 hours.

5. Preheat the oven to 375 degrees. Take out casserole from the fridge while heating the oven. Bake until golden brown, without covering, for 40-50 minutes. Leave to stand before slicing for 5–10 minutes.

Freeze option:

1. Cover the unbaked casserole and ice it. Partially defrost overnight in the refrigerator to use.

2. Take out from the fridge 30 minutes before cooking.

3. Preheat the oven to 375°F. Bake the casserole as instructed, increasing the time required to heat through and read 165°F or the thermometer put in the center.

CHAPTER 8 PORK LAMB & BEEF

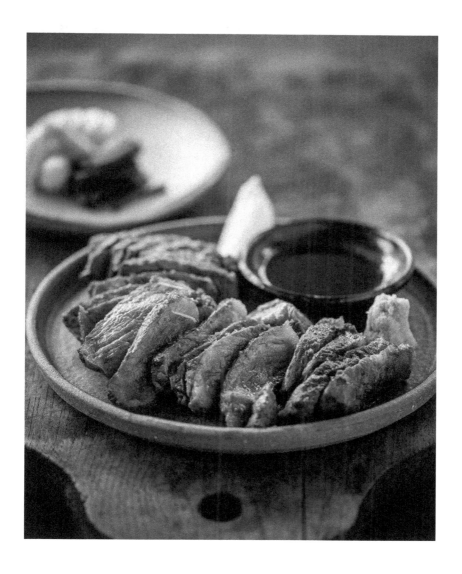

8.1 Meal Prep Slow-Cooker Pork Shoulder

(**Prep. time:** 10hrs | **Servings:** 12 | **Difficulty:** medium)

Serving size: 3 oz.

Per serving: Cal 168, Fat 7g, Carbs 5g, Proteins 21g

Ingredients

- 3 lbs. lean boneless pork shoulder

- 1 tbsp. olive oil

- 1 large yellow onion, sliced

- 10 garlic cloves, sliced

- 1 tsp. cumin

- 1 tsp. paprika

- ¼ cup tomato paste

- ¼ cup coconut amines

- Salt & pepper to taste

Directions

1. Thoroughly dry the pork with a paper towel.

2. Heat the olive oil in a large skillet over moderate to high flame. Add the pork shoulder then cook to brown for 4 min. per side. Remove the shoulder of pork, and put aside.

3. Reduce flame to medium-low under the skillet. Add onion and fry, stirring, for around 2 minutes, until the onion is brown in some areas, & almost charred in others. Add cumin, garlic and paprika. Cook only for around thirty seconds, till fragrant.

4. Put the pork shoulder in a slow cooker and top with the tomato paste. Pour onion, garlic & spices over the pork shoulder and scrape the pan with a rubber spatula. Pour in the coconut amino over the shoulder of pork. Season with salt & pepper. Cover & cook for 8–10 hrs. At low.

5. Shred with 2 forks.

6. Before storage, cool fully. Leftovers can be stored for up to 4 days in an airtight container in the refrigerator, and for up to 3 months in the airtight container in a freezer.

8.2 Grilled Pork Tenderloin

(**Prep. time:** 13 min. | **Servings:** 4 | **Difficulty:** easy)

Serving size: 4 oz.

Per serving: Kcal 141, Fat 4g, Carbs 0g, Proteins 23g

Ingredients

- 1 lb. whole pork tenderloin

- 2 tbsp. Dijon mustard

- Salt and pepper to taste

Directions

1. Preheat to medium-heat, the grill. Cut one gulley right through the middle of pork tenderloin end to end using a paring knife. Be sure to not cut through the entire way. Open and lay the pork flat. Make additional minor cuts to open broader, if necessary.

2. Slather the pork tenderloin on both ends, with Dijon mustard. Sprinkle on both sides, with salt & pepper.

3. Grill five minutes on either side. Remove from grill and cover with foil for 5-10 min. before slicing.

8.3 Chipotle and Cinnamon Baked Pork Chops {one pan meal}

(**Prep. time:** 30 min. | **Servings:** 4 | **Difficulty:** medium)

Serving size: 6 oz. chops + ¾ cup veggies

Per serving: Kcal 141, Fat 4g, Carbs 0g, Proteins 23g

Ingredients

Chipotle Cinnamon Rub:

- 1 tbsp. coconut sugar

- 1 teaspoon of grounded chili powder

- ½ tsp. cinnamon

- ¼ tsp. garlic powder

- ¼ tsp. onion powder

- ¼ tsp. smoked paprika

- Dried oregano, pinch

- ½ tsp. sea salt

- ¼ tsp. grounded black pepper

Pan:

- 2 big carrots (7-8 inch long), cut to half-inch slices

- 2 big parsnips (7-8 inch long), cut to half-inch slices

- 2–3 tbsp. olive oil

- 1.5 lb. boneless loin or pork chops

- Lemon slices, parsley & red chili flakes for garnishing

- Optional: salt & pepper for seasoning each plate

Directions

1. Mix the cinnamon chipotle in a tiny bowl to season. Put aside.

2. Preheat your oven to 400°F. Cut the carrots and parsnips into ½ pieces. Toss the in two tablespoons of olive oil and 2 teaspoons of chipotle cinnamon seasoning.

3. Place the parsnips on the sheet and the carrots flat. Roast in the oven for fifteen minutes.

4. Prepare the pork chops while the vegetable roast.

5. Apply cinnamon chipotle seasoning on each piece of meat. Put each pork chop in a saucepan with one tablespoon of avocado oil or olive oil. Fry the pork for 2-4 min. on medium-high. You have to flip it once.

6. Remove meat from flame & put it with vegetables on a baking pan.

7. Put the pan back into the oven (with pork and vegetables) and bake/roast at 400°F for another 6 to 8 min. or until pork hits 165°F pork internal temperature.

8. Take the pan from the oven and add the garnishes; slices of lemon, flakes of red pepper & fresh parsley.

9. Serve, and have fun.

8.4 Healthy Almond-Crusted Pork Tenderloin

(**Prep. time:** 7 hrs. | **Servings:** 4 | **Difficulty:** medium)

Serving size: 1 g

Per serving: Cal 502, Fat 26g, Carbs 20.3g, Proteins 37.1g

Ingredients

- Pork Tenderloin 1

Marinade:

- Plain Yogurt ¾ cup

- Olive Oil 2 tbsp.

- Minced garlic cloves 2

- Fresh Lemon Juice 1 tbsp.

Crumb Mixture:

- Finely chopped Almonds 1 cup

- Bread Crumbs ½ cup

- Salt and pepper, pinch

Directions

1. Heat the oven until 450

2. Mix marinade mixture together in a small container.

3. Spread the marinade on the pork tenderloin.

4. Put in a dish, covering with saran wrap & allow to rest for 6-24 hours in the refrigerator.

5. Take the meat from the refrigerator & scrape the mixture off.

6. Apply mixture of almonds on the pork and put in a baking dish.

7. Cook 10 min., the tenderloin, and decrease to 275.

8. Bake for another 40-45 min. or till meat reaches 150 internal temperature.

9. Allow to rest for ten min., and slice.

8.5 Vietnamese Brown Rice & Steak Salad

(**Prep. time:** 2 hrs. 20 min. | **Servings:** 8 | **Difficulty:** medium)

Serving size: 1 cup

Per serving: Cal 317, Fat 7.3g, Carbs 48.1g, Proteins 17.6g

Ingredients

- 1 ½ cups + 6 tbsp. brown jasmine rice

- 10 dried small red chilies

- 1 tbsp. canola oil

- 1 lb. trimmed New York strip steak

- ½ tsp. kosher salt

- 6 tbsp. lime juice

- 3 tbsp. fish sauce

- Halved lengthwise & thinly sliced plum tomatoes

- 2 thinly sliced medium shallots

- 1 cup fresh basil leaves

- 1 cup fresh mint leaves

Directions

1. In a medium saucepan, place 1 ½ cups of rice and cover with 2 inches of water. Bring to boil over high flame. Reduce heat to hold a simmer, cover and cook for around 25 minutes until soft. Drain and clean under cold water, till cool.

2. Meanwhile, over medium-high heat, toast chilies in a medium skillet, when fragrant & darkened in places, 2 to 3 min. Shift to mortar or clean spice grinder, then let it cool for around 5 minutes. Grinding the chilies coarsely.

3. Bring the pan back to medium-high heat. Add oil as well as the remaining 6 spoonsful of rice. Cook for about 3 minutes, stirring continuously, till the rice is thoroughly toasted. Scrape onto a paper towel-lined plate to drain & cool, then smash gently in the mortar or with bottom of a large pot. Wipe out the saucepan.

4. Steak with salt to season. Bring the pan back to medium-high heat & add the steak. Cook, flipping once, unless an instant-read thermometer reports medium-rare 130°F, 4 to 5 minutes per side. Put the steak on a clean cutting board and then let it cool down completely, around 25 minutes. Dice the steak.

5. In a large bowl, mix tomatoes, lime juice, fish sauce & shallots, with boiled rice, steak and pinch of ground chilies.

6. Fold it in basil and mint just before eating. Sprinkle with toasted rice, and some ground chili to taste.

CHAPTER 9 DESSERTS

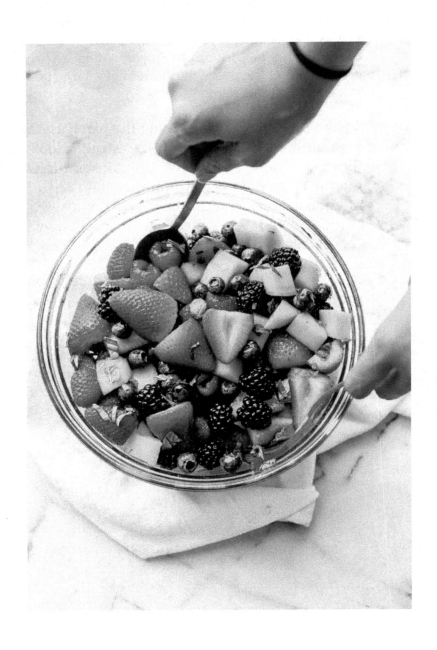

9.1 Berry Fruit Salad with Mangoes

This easy berry fruit salad gives you an inner as well as an outer glow to your complexion! Loaded with a variety of berries, fresh herbs, and a quick and easy dressing!

(**Prep. time:** 10 min. | **Serving:** 5 | **Difficulty:** easy)

Serving size: 1 cup

Per serving: Kcal: 95, Fats: 6g, Carbs: 15g, Proteins: 5g

Ingredients

Dressing:

- 2 tbsp. lemon, freshly squeezed

- 1-2 tbsp. honey

- 1 tbsp. chopped mint

Salad:

- 1 lb. strawberries (hulled and halved)

- 6 oz. each raspberries, blueberries, and blackberries

- 2 mangoes, peeled and diced

- ¼ cup julienned basil

Directions

1. Dressing: In a small container, whisk the honey and lemon together. Use 1 tbsp. of honey as berries and mango are pretty sweet. Use 2 tbsp. if you like it sweeter. Add the mint and mix.

Assembly:

2. Add mangoes and all the berries to a large salad bowl along with basil. Drizzle the salad with the honey dressing and toss until thoroughly mixed.

3. Serve immediately.

9.2 Low-fat Cappuccino Pudding

(**Prep. time:** 1 hr. 10 min. | **Servings:** 5 | **Difficulty:** easy)

Serving size: 1/5 of the recipe

Per serving: Kcal: 204, Fats: 12g, Carbs: 12g, Proteins: 3g

Ingredients

- 1 package 1 oz. instant pudding, vanilla flavored, sugar-free, fat-free

- 2 tsp. instant coffee

- 2 cups fat-free milk, cold

- ⅛ tsp. ground cinnamon

- 1 cup lite cool whip topping, thawed

Directions

1. Mix instant coffee, dry pudding mix, and milk with whisk for 2 minutes.

2. Pour into five dessert bowls.

3. Freeze for 1 hour.

4. Sprinkle cinnamon onto cool whip and mix with a whisk or a spoon and spoon over the pudding before serving!

9.3 No Sugar Apple Pie

An apple pie without the Carbs or sugar, with just the right amount of sweetness to curb your sweet cravings

(**Prep. time:** 1 hr. 10 min. | **Servings:** 8 | **Difficulty:** medium)

Serving size: 1 slice

Per serving: Kcal: 421, Fats: 23g, Carbs: 50g, Proteins: 5g

Ingredients

- $^1/_3$ cup apple juice concentrate, thawed

- Sugar substitute equal to 8 tsp. sugar

- 2 tsp. cornstarch

- 1 tsp. ground cinnamon

- Pie pastry (9 inches), double-crust

- 8 cups tart apples, peeled, thinly sliced

- 1 tbsp. butter

Directions

1. Mix the first four components together.

2. Place pie plate with crust underneath; add apples. Pour the juice mixture over the apples; add the butter.

3. Spread out the remaining pastry to adhere to the top of the pie; cut in the top slits or an apple type. Place over stuffing; flute and seal the edges.

4. Bake for 35 minutes, at 375°F. Raise oven temperature to 400°F; bake for another 15–20 minutes or until apples are soft.

9.4 Frozen Yogurt Fruit Pops

This recipe can be made with any fruit and any flavor of yogurt. Pineapple yogurt with mango chunks or kiwi slices with strawberry yogurt would be delicious. You can also try toppings like roasted coconut or rainbow sprinkles in place of pecans.

(Prep. time: │**Servings:** 12│**Difficulty:** medium)

Serving size: 2 pop

Per serving: Kcal: 55 cal , Fat: 3.5g, Carbs:5g, Proteins: 2g

Ingredients

- ¼ cup pecans, chopped

- 12 cake pop sticks

- ½ cup Greek blueberry yogurt(non-fat)

- 12 strawberries, hulled

- Wax paper

Directions

1. Line a small, wax paper baking sheet. Place on aside.

2. Place the cake pop sticks into the strawberry top. Do not impale into the bottom of the strawberry.

3. In the yogurt, dip each strawberry and shake so that each strawberry is finely covered. When required, use a spoon to help cover the strawberries in yogurt.

4. Garnish 1 tsp. Pecan over each strawberry.

5. Put on the baking sheet, the strawberry pops and freeze for 1–2 hours or until the yogurt is frozen. When frozen, extract the pops from the wax paper and serve or place them in a zip-top bag in a freezer.

9.5 Banana chia pudding

Flax milk and chia seeds make this healthy, creamy dessert a treat!

(Prep. time: 2hrs 10min. | **Servings:** 6 | **Difficulty:** easy)

Serving size: 1/6th of the recipe

Per serving: Kcal: 112, Fats: 5g, Carbs: 20.5g, Proteins: 1.6g

Ingredient

- 1 ½ cups flax milk vanilla-flavored

- 1 large banana, sliced

- 7 tbsp. chia seeds

- 3 tbsp. honey

- 1 tsp. vanilla extract

- ⅛ tsp. sea salt

- Sugar substitute (Splenda or truvia)

Directions

1. Put the milk, banana, chia seeds, sugar substitute, vanilla extract, and sea salt in the respective order; combine until smooth.

2. Measure the mixture into a container, then refrigerate for at least 2 hours until thickened. To eat, put the mixture in small cups.

CONCLUSION

This book came to your hands at the ideal moment. Not only is it a cookbook with the 50 trending recipes that you should know to have new options, but it is also a new tool that you have to surprise your loved ones.

Eating natural, unprocessed foods is the solution for healthy skin, nails, hair, brain, and heart. Only by following the preparations step by step can you achieve your goals.

From now on, you can lose weight, take care of your immune system and give health to those who cook. It is essential that you remember:

1.- This is not a vegan / vegetarian diet.

2.- Experiment with the recipes; put your personal touch.

3.- Do not follow extreme diets; lose weight in a natural way.

4.- It is time to start a new way of eating.